HERBS, HEALTH AND HEALING

How to use the valuable herbals from the heathlands and hedgerows in the treatment of disease as it affects the various systems of the body. Remedies that have been used with success and safety for generations without risk of harmful side effects which are so often attendant on the use of alkaloid derivatives and other suppressive drugs.

D1545387

HERBS, HEALTH
AND HEALING

by
J. HEWLETT-PARSONS D.Sc.

(Founder President and Director of Studies
of The General Council and Register of
Consultant Herbalists)

NATURE'S WAY

THORSONS PUBLISHERS LIMITED
Wellingborough, Northamptonshire

First published 1968
Second Impression 1970
Third Impression 1971
Second Edition (revised and reset) 1975
Second Impression 1977

ISBN 0 7225 0321 0

Typesetting by
Specialised Offset Services Ltd, Liverpool
Made and Printed in Great Britain by
Weatherby Woolnough, Wellingborough,
Northants, England

CONTENTS

INTRODUCTION

Herbal Medicine is the Cinderella of Medicine in this age of suppressive drug monopoly but, like Cinderella, it emerges in the end in all its glory. Unsurpassed in efficacy and in its complete safety in use, after many millenia, it is the salvation of many thousands of chronic cases which as a last and final resort, often in despair, have found new hope and renewed health by the use of some simple herbal.

Today as a result of modern scientific research and analysis we can prove clinically the therapeutic uses of these herbals which have been known empirically over so many generations and used with so much success by so many eminent healers whose names have become a byword in the human story.

The great value of these natural products is that they grow mainly wild in the meadows and the hedgerows and are thus naturally grown and composted products of Nature whose laboratory is without parallel as a supplier of man's most urgent needs. As a result they are rich in the minerals and vitamins as well as other micro-nutrients which enable the body in its particular laboratory to manufacture as and when required all the substances necessary to combat disease in all its forms and manifestations.

Without these vital substances the cell structure of the body is quite unable to produce the many and various antibodies to combat the many armies of infections which beset us. These micro-nutrients which are to be found in these herbals not only give the body the means to cure: they also help to maintain healthy cell structure and so prevent disease and build up immunity to attack.

In this book I have departed from the usual format of listing herbals in alphabetical order with their better known uses and have dealt with the more prominent and specific of them in their most appropriate relationship to the various systems in the human body — and in their application to the treatment of various organic disease conditions.

In this way it will be easy for the reader suffering say from some disorder of the intestines to turn to the chapter on this subject and find for himself the remedy or formula best suited to his own especial needs.

Although this book is presented in a new form and use is made of up-to-date knowledge of the essential micro-nutrient constituents of herbals this is not to say that the findings of the older authorities have been ignored where these are confirmed by modern clinical experiment or supported by proof of efficacy in application. We owe a great debt to those great pioneers in this field commencing with Hippocrates (some

of whose writings are still extant) and following
with our own English Culpeper, Dr Coffin, Dr
Thompson, Fox and a host of others whose
work in the alleviation of human suffering is so
well known among practitioners.

The great advantage of complete herbal
medicines over modern drug treatments is the
fact that the herbalist does not take some
therapeutic agent out of the plant and use it out
of context. It is when this is done that the
harmful side effects are so manifest. The
extraction of quinine from the cinchona bark is
an example of this and there are very many
others.

As they are grown by Nature the herbals
contain a variety of substances in organic
combination and in such proportions as to be
completely compatible with the human body.
They are thus more easily assimilated and
readily available as therapeutic agents in the
body. It is true they will not suppress symptoms
such as pain with the speed of an aspirin tablet
but I can assure my readers that if natural
aspirin is taken in the form it occurs in the
willow tree it will have a far more beneficial and
constructive effect on diseases such as rheumatism (which is what aspirin is prescribed for in
such large quantities by the allopathic profession) and will help the body to attack the cause
of the complaint rather than just alleviating the
pain.

The Circulatory System

The blood stream is often called the 'river of life' and not without reason. It is perhaps the most important system in the human body. It is responsible for conveying nutrition to every part as well as collecting and excreting waste products. The complex compounds for instance in a herbal remedy have first to be broken down by the metabolic processes before they can be distributed to where they may be required for use in a particular organ. This distribution of nutrients as well as herbal therapeutic agents is possible only because of the very tiny blood vessels called capillaries. However, the 'river of life' will not flow at all without an efficient pump and this brings us to —

The Heart

The heart is subject to two kinds of disease — *functional* and *organic*. Of these the organic diseases are by far the most serious in their effect.

Functional disease is usually caused by excesses of various kinds such as alcohol, smoking, etc. The best treatment is to pay attention to the general hygiene — plenty of fresh air and tonics containing natural iron. Of course the excesses must be stopped. One of the best herbals in this field is White Bryony (bryonia) and should be taken regularly as an infusion.

Organic diseases such as pericarditis where the heart action is quicker than normal and where there is palpitation, with tenderness around the heart and difficulty in lying on the left side, are best treated with remedies such as hawthorn. Endocarditis is an inflammation of the lining membrane of the heart caused by rheumatic affections or nephritis. Here the symptoms are palpitation with rapid pulse and there is difficulty in breathing. Warm compresses at night with herbals which are heart sedatives such as Lily of the Valley, is the best treatment for this condition, also for valvular heart disease where the valves have become inflamed or ulcerated and the openings narrowed causing the valve to work inefficiently.

Fatty degeneration of the muscle fibres of the heart is usually caused by faulty nutrition. It is most often found in old people with a history of gout, chronic anaemia and alcoholism. Wheat germ oil and buckwheat are valuable treatments for this condition. The diet must be drastically reformed to include at least one salad meal a day and plenty of fruit while all fried foods and fat meat, etc., should be avoided. One of the finest herbals for this condition is Nux Vomica.

Myocarditis, which can be acute or chronic, is an inflammation of the heart muscle and in its final stages results in fibroid degeneration. Rest and quiet are required in the treatment of this condition with herbals such as Lily of the Valley, Marigold, Hartstongue, Cactus and Tansy.

Heart Remedies

Some indications of herbals useful in specific conditions of the heart have been given. The finest heart nutrient is undoubtedly Hawthorn and for all heart sufferers this is an essential. It can be taken as a food in the form of the fresh hawthorn berry when this is in season. Commence with five berries twice daily after meals and gradually increase by one berry with each dose until a total of 20 berries are being taken per day. Convallaria is similar in action.

The following is a proven and tried herbal formula which is suitable for all conditions which affect the heart:

> 1 oz. Marigold flowers
> 1 oz. Hartstongue
> 1 oz. Tansy
> 1 oz. Vervain
> 1 oz. Valerian root

The ingredients can be obtained in dried form from your Health Food Store or Herbalist. Place them in two pints of boiling water and simmer to 1½ pints. Allow this to cool and then strain, storing in a cool place. Take a wineglassful of the decoction three times daily after meals. This decoction should be freshly made every two or three days.

When the hawthorn berry is not in season the

dried variety can be obtained from your Health Stores or Herbalist and made into a tea infusion or decoction. For this take 2 oz. of the dried berries and simmer in 1½ pints of boiling water until there is approximately one pint left. Allow to cool and strain afterwards, keeping the mixture in a cool place. A wineglassful of this taken at frequent intervals (every two to three hours) will produce wonderful and lasting results for all heart sufferers.

The other heart remedies mentioned can all be prepared as decoctions in the same way. Any of these treatments, once adopted, should be taken over a period of several months.

Disorders of the Blood Vessels and the Circulatory System

A loss of elasticity in the walls of the blood vessels will result in conditions such as blood pressure, varicose veins, chilblains, and haemorrhoids. Obviously if any treatment is to be effective the basic cause of these conditions must first be eradicated before any therapeutic agent will be of real use.

This means that food and remedies which are rich in the nutrients which the body needs to restore and maintain the elasticity of the arterial and venous walls must be incorporated in the daily diet. Foods such as wholemeal bread and wheat germ, buckwheat (which contains rutin) and the citrus fruits which are rich in Vitamin C are essential as well as vegetables such as parsley, leeks and endive.

Since silica and fluorine are the essential minerals required, the herbal remedies which are richest in these will be best for any disorders mentioned above. In this context houndstongue and horsetail are indicated and decoctions made in the same way as those for heart disorders can be made and taken over several months as a basic treatment in conjunction with a sound diet on the lines given.

Treatment for Blood Pressure

Red meat and meat extracts should be avoided in the diet and salads with fruits and vegetables as indicated above should be taken daily. A general mixture would be a combination of the following:

>1 oz. Lime flowers
>1 oz. Yarrow
>1 oz. Uva-ursi
>1 oz. Elder flowers
>1 oz. Scullcap

Place these in 2 pints of boiling water and simmer down to 1½ pints. Allow to cool and strain for use, keeping in a cool storage place. Take a wineglassful of the mixture three or four times daily according to severity of conditions. After meals is preferable for this mixture. As always make this decoction fresh every two or three days. This is an ideal treatment for high blood pressure.

In cases of *low blood pressure* use the following dried herbs:

1 oz. Nettles
1 oz. Marshmallow
1 oz. Kola
½ oz. Wood betony

Prepare this decoction in exactly the same way, adding the herbs to 2 pints of boiling water and simmering down to 1½ pints before cooling and straining ready for use.

Varicose Veins in the Legs

Bandages of extract of Witch Hazel can be worn during sleep at night. Do not bind them too tightly. Just soak the bandage in the extract and place over the area, covering with a dry bandage loosely fastened.

The following mixture should be taken over several months to effect a real improvement in the condition for it must be realized that any treatment for the restoration of elasticity to veins or in fact any tissue will take a long time.

Many years of poor diet, lack of fresh air through improper breathing, etc., are the predisposing factors to these conditions and overnight cures or results cannot be expected:

1 oz. Bayberry bark
1 oz. Wood betony
1 oz. Wood sage
1 oz. Yellow dock
1 oz. Echinacea
1 oz. Boneset

Place these dried prepared herbs (obtainable from your local Registered Medical Herbalist) in 3 pints of boiling water and simmer until you have 2 pints of mixture left. Allow this to cool and then strain and bottle ready for use. Take a wineglassful of this mixture every four hours.

In cases of varicose veins in the testicles (*varicocele*) the same mixture will be found very effective, while the parts can be painted with extract of Witch Hazel every night on retiring.

Haemorrhoids (Piles)

This distressing complaint can be quickly relieved and cleared up with the use of a blend of herbs containing Collinsonin (stone root). Haemorrhoids are really varicose veins occurring in the rectum or at the anus. During the treatment it is imperative that any degree of constipation is avoided and any tendency to liver congestion prevented.

In extreme cases a local application of ointment of Witch Hazel or Nut Gall can be used. The following mixture should be taken for about a month, when all traces of the piles should have disappeared:

      1 oz. Oak bark
      1 oz. Stone root
      1 oz. Black root
      1 oz. Motherwort
      1 oz. Blood root

Place these prepared dried herbs in 2 pints of boiling water and allow to simmer gently until 1½ pints remain. Allow the whole to cool before straining ready for use. Bottle and keep tightly corked in a cool place. Take a wineglassful of the mixture three times daily before meals.

Chilblains

As these usually occur during the winter months and mainly in those with poor circulation it is advisable to take a course of rutin tablets during the early autumn as a preventive measure. The natural rutin tablets are the best, as made from extract of Buckwheat.

It is also essential to make sure that the diet has an adequate amount of foods containing the B group of vitamins and in particular nicotinic acid which is a substance forming part of this vitamin group (wheat germ foods, garlic, leeks, sprouts, etc.). The following mixture of prepared dried herbs made into a decoction is a wonderful treatment:

> 1 oz. Lily of the Valley
> 1 oz. Motherwort
> 1 oz. Scullcap

Simmer these in two pints of boiling water until approximately 1½ pints are left. Cool and strain ready for use. The dose for this mixture is a wineglassful every three hours for about a week. The chilblains can be bandaged with liquid extract of Witch Hazel.

Anaemia

This, apart from being a distressing condition in itself, can also be the cause of such conditions as arthritis later in life. It is a well-known fact that women who have an inadequate diet of natural physiological iron during pregnancy and become anaemic, suffer later in life from arthritis and other allied rheumatic conditions. Some 30 milligrams of iron should be taken in the diet every day for good health.

Here is where the importance of fresh green vegetables comes in. These are rich in easily assimilated iron. Dandelion leaves in the daily salad are especially useful and white fish is one of the best sources of iron which in this form is again easily assimilable by the body.

For those suffering from anaemia the following mixture will be found very reliable and it will readily rectify the condition if the rules mentioned in respect of diet are also observed:

1 oz. Blue cohosh
1 oz. Tansy
¾ oz. Black cohosh
½ oz. Aloes barb

These dried herbs should be simmered in 2 pints of boiling water until a residue of 1½ pints remains, after which the mixture should be cooled and strained ready for use. A wineglassful is taken every three hours between meals. Again the mixture, as in the case of all these decoctions, should be prepared fresh every two or three days and in this instance it should be taken regularly over a period of about two months for the best results.

Diseases of the Digestive System

Dyspepsia or indigestion in the sense of imperfect gastric digestion is one of our most common ailments and results from many disorders of the stomach of a functional and structural nature. The symptoms can be quite serious and some combinations of these are especially characteristic of gastric disease. Some of them are due to fermentative changes in indigestible or undigested food. The products may be gaseous when they will cause flatulent distension or they may cause pain by directly irritating the mucous membrane.

Irritation of the membrane of any part of the digestive tract can be the cause of catarrh with the consequent pain and other allied symptoms of gastritis. In the more chronic cases the pain may be due to an ulcer, further irritated by food or gastric juice where the balance of the secretion is disturbed. Pain may be felt at the 'pit of the stomach' or around the left side or through the trunk to the back.

There is no doubt that the pain and discomfort is caused in the immediate sense by spasm or increased peristalsis excited by these causes. All this can so easily lead to nausea and vomiting which are indicative of gastric disturbance. When there is much vomiting, bile often regurgitates from the duodenum into the stomach and is then vomited.

We are all familiar with the terms heartburn and waterbrash which are applied to a burning sensation in the stomach area. This happens in dyspepsia and is often accompanied by regurgitation of fluid which can be felt as high up as the pharynx. Ulcer sufferers can, over a period of years, have recurring attacks of haematosis (bleeding).

Herbal remedies offer a wide range of healing powers in all affections of the digestive system and those with the widest range of therapeutic action are Comfrey, Coltsfoot (as good for catarrh of the stomach as for the respiratory system), Slippery Elm, and Marshmallow.

Acute Gastric Catarrh

The usual cause is irritation of the stomach caused by foods which are either unsuitable or have been eaten in excessive quantities. Surplus foods which the body cannot handle undergo decomposition producing substances which irritate the mucous membranes. It can happen to people of all ages. Unripe or overripe fruit is a common cause in children when a bilious attack is the result. Quite often there can be serious constipation attendant on acute gastric catarrh. When this is the case a warm enema of an infusion of Slippery Elm bark should be administered.

One of the finest foods for eliminating

inflammation of the digestive tract is pineapple juice. The juice has an affinity for membranes of all types and is said to even dissolve the membrane of Dyptheria. Certainly one or two days on a fast taking only pineapple juice is a splendid beginning to any herbal treatment for this complaint. After this the patient can take a light diet of Slippery Elm food (obtainable from Health Food Stores) steamed fish and milk.

The finest herbal mixture is as follows, using dried herbs:

      1 oz. Comfrey
      1 oz. Clivers
      1 oz. Meadowsweet
      1 oz. Marshmallow

Simmer in 2 pints of boiling water until about 1½ pints are left. Allow to cool and strain. Take a wineglassful of the mixture every four hours for the first few days and afterwards three times daily after meals.

Chronic Gastric Catarrh

This can result from untreated acute gastric catarrh or from excessive consumption of tea, alcohol, iced drinks, etc., or incomplete mastication of food. In these chronic cases the first essential is to give the whole alimentary tract a complete rest. This means abstinence from all those artifical and denatured food products which are such irritants to the membranes lining the alimentary canal. Try an initial fast of two or three days (according to general condition) on unsweetened pineapple juice. The ideal is the juice of the fresh fruit although in this country fresh pineapples are packed before they are ripe and are thus short of that complete solar radiation which makes the best fruit. The unsweetened juice can be obtained in tins and it has been found that the juice extracted from Hawaiian pineapples or those from Trinidad are best.

Follow the two or three day fast with a light, balanced diet consisting of fresh raw leafy and root vegetables, wholewheat bread and whole-grain cereals, bran etc. In this way the membranes will be cleansed and re-toned. The two day fast on pineapple juice may be undertaken once a week until the condition has made some real improvement.

The best herbal mixture for these chronic cases is to take the following dried herbs:

1 oz. Black horehound
1 oz. Coltsfoot
1 oz. Calumba
1 oz. Comfrey
½ oz. Raspberry
½ oz. Marshmallow

Simmer in 2½ pints of boiling water until about 2 pints are left. Cool and strain for use. The dose is a wineglassful every three or four hours for the first few days and then three times daily after meals until the condition has completely cleared up.

Peptic Ulcer
It is thought that the acute variety of this

complaint occurs mainly in women between 20 and 30 while the chronic variety is more prevalent in males of middle age. There is always a risk of haemorrhage. However, many cases are known to recover after safe herbal treatment in a few weeks.

Naturally diet is very important here and again a diet of fish and milk is the ideal with Slippery Elm food made as a breakfast cereal taken each morning and as a night-cap. Since pineapple juice contains a substance very like pepsin and has the property of being able to partially digest certain types of protein food this too is an essential part of the diet in these cases. A wineglassful of the fruit juice should be taken regularly before every meal, especially when protein foods are to be eaten.

The best herbal treatment is the following in the form of dried herbs made into a decoction:

1½ oz. Comfrey
1½ oz. Marshmallow
1 oz. Meadowsweet
1 oz. Yellow dock

The whole is placed in 2½ pints of boiling water and simmered until about 2 pints are left. After cooling, the mixture is strained ready for use. A wineglassful every three hours is taken for the first two weeks of treatment and then every four hours for a further three weeks or until cure is effected.

The Intestines

Disturbances of the large and small intestine can

have many and various causes and space precludes an exhaustive preamble into the many primary factors which may result in one or more distressing symptoms making themselves felt. In fact, in some cases the cause can be of purely nervous origin. Some of the more common complaints are dealt with here and the best possible herbal treatment given. It is well to remember that as with stomach disorders, diet can be one of the predisposing factors in all these complaints and a serious appraisal should be made of this at the outset of any treatment if there is to be any cure.

Certainly our popular present day diets of stodgy food in the form of refined starches and sugars and the over-indulgence in food generally are the biggest evils of our time. The sooner a preventive attitude to disease is adopted by the acceptance of a sane rational diet which provides an adequate intake of all the vital nutrients without the irritations of denatured, refined and otherwise useless foodstuffs, the better it will be for all of us.

Diarrhoea

This condition may indeed be due purely to a nervous cause, or it may be due to over-stimulation by bad foodstuffs or drugs. Quite often undigested food is passed which so irritates the membrane as to cause the diarrhoea. An enema is often a great help at the outset of treatment and our good friend Slippery Elm bark taken as a food made with milk is invaluable. Arrowroot is also very useful and can be made into a food with milk. The best herbal mixture is made from the following dried herbs:

1 oz. Oak bark
1 oz. Tormentilla
1 oz. Bistort

simmered for 20 minutes in 1 pint of boiling water. Cooled and strained. The mixture to be taken one wineglassful every two hours until the symptoms abate.

Constipation

Sedentary habits, and an over-abundance of refined and denatured starches and sugars in the diet are the predisposing factors in this condition. It can also result from stomach disorders and sometimes from psychological factors. The first essential is the adoption of a sound balanced diet which will not only help physiologically but which will also bring about a mental uplift and an optimism which will form the basis of cure.

All white bread, white sugars, and their products such as chocolate, sweets, cakes, etc. should be ruthlessly removed from the daily dietary. In their place wholewheat bread, honey, with bulk foods such as brain and raw leafy vegetables such as cabbage, lettuce, endive etc. should be eaten to aid normal peristalsis. Fresh fruit should be taken after every meal instead of the inevitable cup of coffee or tea.

If the following decoction is also prepared and taken with these instructions any sufferer from ordinary constipation should find an encouraging improvement in the condition in a very short time.

    1 oz. Black root
    1 oz. Echinacea
    1 oz. Gentian

Simmer these for 20 minutes in 3 pints of boiling water. Cool and strain. The dose is a tumblerful of the mixture before meals.

Catarrhal Enteritis

This is inflammation of the mucous membrane of the bowel caused by the use of violent purgatives, unripe fruit, perhaps a chill in hot weather, etc. Diarrhoea is the principal symptom, with griping pains. A decoction is made from the following dried herbs:

    1 oz. Elder flowers
    1 oz. Burdock
    1 oz. Peppermint
    1 oz. Golden rod
    1 oz. Red clover

Simmer gently in 2 pints of boiling water for 20 minutes. Cool and strain. Take a wineglassful of the mixture every two hours until the condition has eased. It will be found an ideal remedy.

Mucous Colitis

The main symptom of this disease is the discharge from the rectum of tough mucus which looks like bowel casts. It occurs most often in neurotic types. A very good herbal mixture is made as follows. Take the following dried herbs:

  1 oz. Marshmallow
  1 oz. Collinsonin (stone root)
  1 oz. Red clover
  1 oz. Raspberry leaves

Simmer these gently in 2 pints of boiling water for 20 minutes, allow to cool and then strain for use. The dose is a wineglassful of the mixture after each meal.

Appendicitis

At the caecum or blind end of the large intestine is a small worm-like projection called the appendix. The removal of this when inflamed (appendectomy) became very popular in this country following its removal from King Edward VII at the beginning of this century. There is no doubt that many a healthy appendix has been removed since that time and that many cases of inflammation (appendicitis) which could have been easily curable by other means were treated by willing surgeons on willing victims who thought they suffered from a very socially acceptable complaint and took the 'royal' road to recovery.

The late Dr Havelock Ellis, who died in the mid-thirties at an advanced age, stated in his autobiography that at intervals throughout his life he had suffered from the symptoms which in later years he came to know as appendicitis. He wrote that when these symptoms became acute all he did was to go to bed for a few days on a light diet when the symptoms invariably cleared up and he resumed his normal working life. He died with his appendix intact. It does seem certain that many more patients have died from post operative peritonitis than have ever died as a result of appendicitis.

Symptoms: Appendicitis usually attacks at intervals with periods of complete freedom from the symptoms between. In the usual attacks the victim feels sick with pain of a griping nature round the navel or in the right side of the abdomen. The symptoms of constipation or diarrhoea may also be present and the whole area of that part of the abdomen is very sensitive to the touch, while there is a rise in temperature with a rapid pulse.

It quite often happens during pregnancy in women with a tendency to digestive disturbances. It can also be the result of gastric or duodenal ulcer or inflammation of the gall-bladder, but the actual cause would seem to be a mystery. It has been put down at various times to germs such as streptococci, etc.

Treatment: It will be seen from the above how important is attention to general health and particularly the health of the alimentary tract. Too much stress cannot be placed upon a soundly balanced diet. There is no doubt at all that a good deal of suffering due to inflammation of various parts of the alimentary tract and the digestive system generally is due to the almost pathological consumption of denatured sugar products among the inhabitants of the so-called civilized countries of the Western

World. We in the British Isles tend to be the worst offenders, according to the latest statistics, and the sugar consumption per head in Britain is simply appalling.

If any treatment for appendicitis is to have any hope of success it cannot be emphasised too strongly that eating habits must be drastically reformed on Nature Cure lines. This means the total abstention from all denatured white flour and white sugar and their products, and a very frugal intake of sugar of any kind (even raw Barbados sugar) and wholemeal flour and bread. All pastry, cakes, biscuits and such-like useless foodstuffs must be completely and totally cut out of any diet.

Concentrate on a diet of fresh whole foods consisting in the main of fresh raw salads, baked jacket potatoes (for starch) and a preponderance of fresh raw fruits. Do not over-work the stomach and digestive system with too frequent eating. Take only two main meals each day and make the breakfast a very light meal of fresh fruit. In this way can a safe and permanent cure be expected. Naturally if there is any doubt at all about the severity or the emergency of the condition the advice and services of a skilled practitioner should be sought immediately.

Fortunately the herbalist has some wonderful remedies for appendicitis and indeed some miraculous cures have been achieved by the use of iris tenax in homoeopathic doses. Anyone suffering from attacks of appendicitis is recommended to obtain homoeopathic powders of iris tenax. These should be obtained in two potencies: six powders of the potency CM and six powders of the potency 30.

While adopting a diet as outlined above and after having spent two days on an exclusive diet of pineapple juice taken at frequent intervals during the day, using about three pints each day (with an enema each morning of this two-day fruit juice treatment) the patient can proceed with the powders.

On the first morning after the pineapple juice treatment and on commencement of a sound diet, take one of the CM potency powders. On alternate days thereafter, and until the six powders are used, take one of the 30 potency powders. Following this take one of the CM powders at monthly intervals until the remaining five powders of this potency have been used up. These powders can be obtained from Nelson and Co. Homoeopathic Chemists, 73 Duke Street, off Oxford Street, London, W.1. Many homoeopathic practitioners regard this iris tenax treatment as a specific in the cure of appendicitis.

A very valuable herbal mixture which can be made up at home and which can be taken for about a month is as follows. Take these dried prepared herbs:

> 2 oz. Comfrey root
> 1 oz. Avena sativa (oats)
> 1 oz. Golden seal

Simmer these in three pints of boiling water until 1½ pints remain. Cool and strain. Take a wineglassful of this mixture after every meal.

Worms

The tapeworm, roundworm and threadworm are the most common in man and there are many herbs which are effective in their eradication. These include wormwood, garlic, male fern, tansy, etc. It is best to obtain the fluid extract of any of these from your local Registered Herbalist and take the recommended dose. An enema of garlic juice is also very helpful.

Diseases of the Skin

The skin is in reality a very important part and organ of the body. It is at the same time part of the respiratory system and an organ of elimination. It mirrors the general condition of the body. It is inconceivable to have a healthy skin covering an unhealthy body. It protects the body, regulates the body temperature, eliminates body waste and assists in respiration.

Usually skin diseases are not in reality local conditions but are external manifestations of deeper underlying conditions present in one or more organs or parts of the body. For example, it can be readily understood when it is realized that the skin is a breathing apparatus that when asthma is suppressed by drug treatment it is quite unusual for the victim of such treatment to quickly manifest symptoms of eczema in the skin. In other words the skin has attempted to take over the intolerable burden from its close partner, the lungs.

Thus the general approach to all skin diseases should be attention to general health. Cleansing of the alimentary tract by frequent short fasts, colonic irrigations or enemas, adoption of good breathing exercises with plenty of healthy exercise designed to improve the circulation and increase metabolism.

Skin Lesions

Skin disease manifests through many and various lesions such as macules which are spots or stains on the skin due to pigmentation as in freckles or after haemorrhage. Papules or pimples which are small (like pinheads), are hard elevations of the skin. Vesicles are small blisters with fluid content such as occur in herpes zoster, etc. Blebs are much larger blisters than vesicles. They may have a serous or blood content. Pustules are like vesicles except that their contents are purulent.

Ulcers or sores are suppurations and when they heal scars are left. These are fibrous tissue in which true skin is absent. Fissures are chaps or cracks in the skin caused by loss of elasticity. Scales consist of masses of epithelial cells which are thrown off in certain diseases. The skin can also manifest scabs or crusts made up of dried secretion of a serous or bloody nature. All these signs and symptoms can be recognized in various skin disorders but again it must be emphasized that the general health must be looked to as well as the treatment of the actual skin condition if lasting cure is to be obtained.

Pruritis

This disorder is mainly functional and may occur generally or locally. There are usually no visible symptoms other than perhaps the effect of scratching by the patient. The main characteristic is itching of the skin with no visible cause. When it is general it can be a symptom of jaundice. During treatment of this complaint a saltless diet should be adhered to and all spices and pickles, etc., discontinued. Lactic oats taken every day are useful in the diet.

A tea made with Horsetail is a wonderful remedy or 1 oz. of each of the following dried herbs: Parsley, Yarrow, Olives, Marshmallow and Witch Hazel simmered from two pints to 1½ pints of water. Cool, strain and take a wineglassful every three hours. A local application of chickweed ointment as well as cold compresses is also very useful.

Blackheads

This unsightly condition which often afflicts the adolescent is again often due to a too fatty diet. A lotion of lemon and Witch Hazel is very useful in clearing up the blackheads while a decoction made of the following dried herbs is also helpful:

> 1 oz. Figwort
> 1 oz. Turkey corn
> 1 oz. Echinacea
> 1 oz. Thuja
> 1 oz. Yellow dock
> ½ oz. Arctium lappa
> ½ oz. Iris versicolor

Simmer in 2 pints of boiling water until 1½ pints are left. Cool and strain. A wineglassful every four hours is the dose. The taking of sugar will aggravate this condition.

Acne

Another unsightly complaint which chiefly affects the face (nose and forehead) shoulders and upper part of the chest. It is apparently caused by a bacillus which causes the pustular eruption, though there may be a secondary inflammation caused by staphylococci. Again this usually attacks those between the ages of 12 and 25 and is associated with adolescence.

Outward applications are useless for this condition as a general rule although hot Epsom salts baths twice weekly have been found very beneficial. For these, use the cheaper variety of Commercial Epsom salts obtainable from most chemists in 7 lb bags. Dissolve half this quantity in a bath of water as hot as can be comfortably borne and relax in the bath commencing with a maximum duration of five to seven minutes. Dry thoroughly and retire at once.

With each succeeding bath increase the time until a maximum of 15 minutes has been reached. Do not use soap with these baths as this will inhibit the therapeutic action of the salts.

Ultra-violet treatment is very beneficial for this complaint but this should be taken only under expert supervision.

All sugars and starches should be precluded from the diet, as well as all forms of alcohol and cheese, except cottage cheese. The main thing is to aim at a diet of lean meat, fresh fish (steamed), yogurt, buttermilk, and an abundance of fresh green and root vegetable salads with about 2 lb of fresh fruit daily.

The best herbal mixture is made from the following dried herbs:

1 oz. Figwort
2 oz. Echinacea
1½ oz. Thuja
1 oz. Rumex crispus
1 oz. Iris versicolor

These dried herbs should be placed in 2 pints of boiling water and simmered until 1½ pints are left. Cool and strain for use. Take a wineglassful of the mixture every four hours and make fresh supplies every two or three days. This treatment may take a month or so for best results.

Psoriasis

This is a very distressing condition which can affect the whole body including the scalp. It usually commences at the elbows and knees. Scales of a silvery character form as an overgrowth of the skin and the deeper layers of the epidermis are affected. There is great irritation with an irresistible urge to scratch. The skin often cracks and bleeds. It is claimed that this disease is often the result of tuberculosis in a previous generation, usually two generations back.

A very high potency dose of Homoeopathic baccilinum (200) given initially will often commence improvement. Powders of bacillinum 200 can be obtained from Nelson and Co., Homoeopathic Chemists of Duke Street, London, W.1.

An all chicken diet has been known to

completely eradicate this disease when combined with a suitable herbal treatment. Certainly treatment for this condition must be aimed at the whole body and to do this it is best to commence with a fast of three or four days on grapefruit or orange juice, taking an enema each morning of the fast.

The affected areas should be painted every night with fluid extract of Blood Root which can be obtained from any Registered Medical Herbalist or from a good Health Food Store or Herbalists' supplier. In this case also, ultra-violet light treatment has been found to alleviate, though it is not a cure. During the summer months the sufferer should sunbathe as much as possible. Never apply soap to the body, particularly the affected areas as this will certainly aggravate the condition.

The best herbal formula for psoriasis is to use dried herbs as follows:

    3 oz. Jamaica sarsaparilla
    1 oz. Mezereon
    1 oz. Guaacum
    1 oz. Yellow dock
    1 oz. Burdock
    1 oz. American bittersweet elm
    1 oz. Black elder flowers
    1 oz. Mandrake
    1 oz. Fumitory
    1 oz. Wood sanicle

Simmer gently for four hours in 4 quarts of water. Cool and then strain. Add a further 2 quarts of water and simmer again for the same length of time. Cool again and then strain carefully. Now add 1 oz. of Queen's Delight, Prickly Ash and Sassafras. Simmer this for a further hour and again cool and strain ready for use. Keep this wonderful decoction in a cool place, or in a fridge, and take a wineglassful four times daily between meals.

Eczema

This can be chronic or acute and as mentioned in the introduction can be closely associated with asthma. It is accompanied by irritation and can manifest several of the various lesions which were mentioned at the beginning of this chapter such as papules, vesicles and pustules. It is a non-contagious disease and there is usually a great deal of inflammation present. It happens to people of all ages but men are more susceptible than women as a rule.

The skin of course loses its elasticity, becoming thicker than normal and quite often there is a serious discharge which can become purulent (pus). This when it dries forms crusts. There are several types which come under the common heading of Eczema: that caused by constant contact with some allergy such as mineral oil or grease which is then occupational; that due to foods to which the patient may be allergic such as eggs or cheese; that due to general metabolic disturbances; that due to a purely nervous cause, and lastly there is that caused by parasite or other infection.

The treatment, as for psoriasis, must be of a

general nature and the general health of the whole body must be improved by general body cleansing treatments. The three or four day fast with enemas is a good beginning with hot Epsom salts baths as described for acne.

Plenty of fresh air and sunlight is essential for improvement to take place. An all fruit diet is also a good sequel to the fast, occupying a further week before a diet of fresh salads, fruit and a very limited quantity of wholemeal bread, etc., is adopted. Outward applications of poultices or Marshmallow leaves or pulverized Marshmallow root and Slippery Elm can follow the hot Epsom salts bath and these are best left on all night. Cold Epsom salts compresses are also very useful in allaying the irritation.

The following herbal formula should be commenced as soon as the fast and the fruit diet has been concluded. Take the following dried herbs:

> 2 oz. Echinacea
> 2 oz. Thuja
> 2 oz. Yellow dock
> 2 oz. Burdock
> 1 oz. Parsley piert
> 1 oz. Uva ursi
> 1 oz. Clivers
> 1 oz. Gentian
> 1 oz. Gravel root
> 1 oz. Wild carrot
> 1 oz. Nettles
> 1 oz. Blue flag

Simmer these slowly in six pints of water for

two hours. Allow to cool, and strain for use. Always keep in a cool place. The dose is a wineglassful of the mixture every three to four hours according to whether the symptoms are acute or chronic.

Seborrhoea

This is a functional disorder of the oil glands of the skin when an abnormal amount of sebum is secreted. It is common in the scalp and in a few cases may spread down the face to the limbs and trunk. It occurs mostly during puberty or adolescence. It is unpleasant in that it can give off an unpleasant odour due to decomposition of the sebaceous matter, especially when it occurs under the prepuce.

Fats should be restricted in the diet to vegetable oils and a very limited amount of whole cereals should be taken. Otherwise the instructions regarding an abundance of fresh fruit and vegetable salads should be followed. The best herbal treatment is to take 1 oz. each of the following dried herbs: Echinacea, Thuja, Burdock, Blue Flag and Queen's Delight and simmer them in 3 pints of water for about two hours. Cool and strain, taking a wineglassful of the mixture after every meal. The affected areas should be bathed with a lotion of liquid extract of Witch Hazel.

Diseases of the Respiratory System

It is not possible in a small manual such as this to deal with the more serious chest and lung diseases such as chronic bronchitis, emphysema, and the many others such as asthma. In these cases it is recommended that the sufferer seek the advice and expert help of a Registered Medical Herbalist.

However, it is well to note than a great many of these diseases are avoidable and there would be a lot less incidence of them if attention was paid to diet and general health, thus preventing and avoiding the necessity of cure. It is true that statistics prove that in our modern cities with their ever increasing traffic, which results in such air pollution, these more serious lung conditions are more prevalent.

Governments all over the world are at last waking up to the increasing dangers of air pollution by petrol and diesel fumes as well as those resulting from coal combustion, and from factory chimneys, etc. The Clean Air Act in England has done something to mitigate this latter menace but the dangers from oil and petrol fumes go unchecked. The best advice to city dwellers whose lives are spent for the most part in these undesirable atmospheres is to get out into the fresh country or coastal air as often as possible.

The one day a week bumper-to-bumper trek from the city to the coast is not the answer as by far the most part of the time is spent in driving in an even more confined atmosphere of diesel and petrol fumes than when free in the city itself. The habit of smoking is worst of all when indulged in such an atmosphere and it is hardly to be wondered that in these circumstances this can be the straw which breaks the camel's back.

The following pages of this chapter will be confined to dealing with the more common afflictions of the respiratory tract but in dealing with these we must not forget that the chronic diseases mentioned above will all yield to expert herbal treatment when attention is also paid to the general health and way of life of the patient. Here diet is of the utmost importance as is exercise and good breathing to a regular rhythm. There are many useful handbooks on the very valuable Yoga systems of breath control which can be recommended to every sufferer of chronic respiratory affections.

One of the best breathing exercises is to stand by an open window every morning on rising and spend five minutes breathing in slowly, counting up to the limit of inhaling. Hold the breath for twice this count and breath out in four times the count. This can be repeated before retiring and it will be found to induce good sound sleep in those who find it difficult to get off after the day's stress and strain.

Treatment: In all cases of lung conditions the blood and nerves must be considered as well as the symptoms of the condition. For this reason the regular breathing as outlined above is a 'must' during the treatment of all the conditions mentioned here and no herbal or other treatment will ever be satisfactory until the patient has learned to control breathing to some extent.

As the great teachers of Yoga will affirm, good rhythmic breathing not only has a physiological effect but it also affects in a beneficial way the nerves and the blood. What the Eastern sages call 'Prana' or Life Force is intimately linked with good rhythmic breathing and every inhalation results in an intake of this 'Prana' as well as air. It is vital therefore when following treatment for any of the following common conditions to adopt a system of rhythmic breathing and thus prevent the necessity for ever having to seek treatment for the more serious lung conditions.

Chronic Nasal Catarrh

For this condition the Herbalist can offer some wonderful remedies which have stood the test of many centuries. They are non-suppressive and with the help of a good diet and breathing exercises will attack the cause and not just alleviate the symptoms. In the initial stages of treatment a nasal douche of one or two drops of eucalyptus oil in four drops of olive oil can be used.

Take the following dried herbs:

1 oz. Boneset
1 oz. Ragwort
1 oz. Burdock
1 oz. Cascara
1 oz. Clivers
1 oz. Golden rod

Simmer in 3 pints of water for an hour. Cool and strain. Take a wineglassful of the mixture after every meal.

Hay Fever
Sometimes this is the result of a neurotic personality or it may result from an allergy to pollen floating in the atmosphere. It is known also to run in families. This is another condition in which the general health must be taken in hand and a sound balanced diet adopted of good salad meals with plenty of fruit, and a minimum of starch and sugars. The mixture outlined for nasal catarrh is also suitable for this condition.

Golden Seal
Some readers who have a knowledge of herbal medicine may well wonder why little mention has been made of this wonderful remedy so far. It deserves special mention on its own account but as it is expensive to buy it has been omitted from most treatments already given. However, it is by far the most wonderful remedy the Herbalist has to use whenever a membrane of any kind in the body is involved.

Conditions of the stomach, the intestines, and lungs and bronchii are all regions of the body for which this famous remedy has a predilection. It can be used alone as an infusion or decoction of the root or in conjunction with other remedies added to further enhance its value. 1 oz. of the root, simmered in a pint of water for an hour and allowed to cool, can be taken between meals a wineglassful at a time in addition to any of the mixtures already mentioned for conditions affecting any of the membranes of the body. It should be taken between meals about every three hours.

For ulcerated conditions of membranes it is unsurpassed — conditions like duodenal ulcer, ulcerated colitis, chronic bronchitis, etc. In fact whenever there is mucus. The following formula is one of the best: take the following dried herbs:

> 1 oz. Golden seal (Hydrastis)
> 1 oz. Cranesbill
> 1 oz. Marshmallow root
> ½ oz. Echinacea
> ½ oz. Phytolacca

Simmer in 3 pints of boiling water for two hours. Cool and strain. Take a wineglassful of the mixture every three hours.

Coughs, Colds and Influenza

These are usually annual visitors which are responsible for a great deal of lost time in the working year. Whenever the onset of a cold or chill is felt take to a light diet with plenty of pineapple juice. A tea made with dried Elder flowers and Peppermint on going to bed will often 'nip in the bud' a threatened cold. If a cough develops this can be quickly soothed by the following mixture:

1 oz. Ground ivy
1 oz. Horehound
1 oz. Hyssop
1 oz. Honey

Simmer in 1 pint of water for an hour. Cool and strain. Take a tablespoonful frequently until the cough has subsided.

One of the finest remedies for coughs and bronchial affections is to chop up a Spanish Onion in a small dish or saucer and cover with honey. Cover this with another plate or dish and leave overnight. In the morning strain off the liquor and take a teaspoonful frequently. It can have miraculous results in the most stubborn of coughs.

Ground Ivy and Horehound with Hyssop as in the above formula are also wonderful in action and no-one should neglect this remedy who suffers from any kind of affection of the respiratory tract.

Diseases of the Nervous System

How often have we heard the expression — 'Oh it's my nerves', and certainly we live in an age when the stresses and strain of our way of life tend to have an increasingly deleterious effect on our nerves. Only by well ordered lives with self discipline can we hope to withstand the many and various inducements which lead to indulgences which are conducive to ill health, particularly involving the nervous systems of the body.

Lesions in the motor sensory nervous system can lead to muscle cramps, spasms and even paralysis. For these conditions the Herbalist has a species of plant known as the primula to help. This includes varieties of the Primrose and the Cowslip. Wood Betony enhances the action of the Primrose. Primrose is also a wonderful remedy for sleeplessness.

In fact, for all cases where muscle spasm is present and for insomnia as well as muscular rheumatism, take 2 oz. of one or other variety of Primrose or Cowslip and 1 oz. of Wood Betony and simmer in 2 pints of water for one hour. Cool and strain, afterwards taking a wineglassful of the mixture every three to four hours according to the severity of the condition.

The Primrose

The German name for this gives us a much better idea as to its therapeutic character. It is Schluesselkey which means 'Keyflower'. Being a spring flower it is associated in ancient lore with renewed vital force or vitality. It can always be relied on to produce good results as a sedative and an anti-spasmodic. It is a very useful remedy in cerebral congestion, stroke, neuralgia and migraine as well as rheumatism of the muscular and gouty types.

Neuritis

This can involve one or several nerves and can be acute or chronic. There is inflammation of the nerve sheaths or nerve fibres. Diet which is rich in foods containing all the vitamin B group is essential. Yeast taken daily is a great help to supplement the diet. A very good herbal mixture can be made by taking the following dried herbs:

> 1 oz. Mistletoe
> 1 oz. Scullcap
> 1 oz. Lupulin
> 1 oz. Gentian
> 1 oz. Valerian

Simmer in 3 pints of water for one hour. After cooling, strain and take a wineglassful of the mixture three times daily after meals.

Neuralgia

This is usually aggravated by debility, anaemia or other run down general conditions. It may be due to irritation of a nerve such as in tooth decay or it may be the result of neuritis. For this condition the best herbal treatment is to make a mixture of the following dried herbs:

2 oz. Scullcap
2 oz. Lupulin
1 oz. Asafoetida
1 oz. Gentian
½ oz. Valerian

Simmer in 4 pints of water until about 3 pints are left. Cool and strain. Take a wineglassful of the mixture every three hours.

Nervous Shock

As a first treatment after accidents or in times of severe mental strain as in the event of bad news, etc., Arnica is a wonderful remedy. As this plant taken as a plain tea or decoction can be a violent irritant and is poisonous, it should only be taken in Homoeopathic form. It is best to get powders of the 12x potency.

Neurasthenia

Nervous exhaustion or neurasthenia is often the result of overwork, prolonged anxiety, worry or emotional shock. It can result from abuse of the body by alcohol, etc. Sexual neurasthenia is also common, resulting in loss of sexual desire and impotence. In general cases there is also loss of muscular power.

Rest and a diet rich in nutrients of the nervous system is necessary if treatment is to be a success. The best herbal mixture for these cases is made up of the following dried herbs:

    2 oz. Wild yam
    1 oz. Valerian
    1 oz. Gentian root
    1 oz. Scullcap
    1 oz. Mistletoe

Simmer in 4 pints of water until 3 pints are left. Allow to cool and strain, taking a wineglassful of the mixture every three hours.

Diseases of the Liver and Gall-Bladder

The liver is a solid dark brown coloured organ and the largest gland in the body. It weighs on average about 3½ lb and has dimensions of about 12 in. across with a thickness of about 6 in. at its maximum. Situated in the right side of the abdominal cavity the top part of it is rounded in shape to enable it to fit into the cavity of the diaphragm where it rests on the other organs of the abdomen. It has several functions, being an organ of excretion as well as secreting substances like bile.

The blood supply to the liver is carried via the hepatic artery and the portal vein near to which are the hepatic ducts. These join to form the very short single duct which then connects with the cystic duct which is attached to the gall-bladder. It is through this system of complicated ducts that the bile manufactured in the liver is carried for storage in the gall-bladder. The cystic duct also joins with the hepatic duct to form the common bile-duct and this opens into the small intestine so that bile may also be carried directly to the small intestine.

The liver is also vital to the nourishment of the body and is a great repository of nutrients. Whenever the body is in urgent need of energy the liver will go to work and manufacture the energizing substances required by the body for digested foods, especially the sugars and the starches.

If the diet is badly balanced and then are excesses of various foods eaten, the liver will not function at its best. This is also true if not enough exercise is taken. A healthy liver can only be maintained by a good sound diet and plenty of exercise to keep it in top condition. Upsets in the liver caused by strain on its delicately balanced functions will cause a variety of diseases such as cirrhosis, indigestion and diseases of the gall-bladder. An upset condition of the bile-ducts will cause jaundice. In fact, indigestion can be a symptom of diseases of the liver and gall-bladder or of the kidneys, appendix, heart or even the lungs.

Cirrhosis of the Liver
This can be caused by the intake of too much alcohol or, in cases where the diet is rich, in spicy foods such as curries, which is why it is a common complaint among the Hindus. Sometimes the bacteria which are harmless in the intestines make their way to the liver and set up an infection which becomes chronic, causing cirrhosis. In this condition the liver shrinks and a hard knobbly surface is formed. The disease is more common in men than in women and in middle-aged men in particular. The symptoms are discomfort in the pit of the stomach with sickness and vomiting. There is often insomnia

and the symptoms of dropsy, while the urine becomes scanty and thick.

This is a case when meat should not be eaten and a light fish diet should be adopted with plenty of fresh green salads and fruit. The lemon and grapefruit are particularly valuable, while the orange is a fruit which must be left severely alone. Naturally no alcoholic drinks of any kind should be taken. Treatment for this condition should always be commenced with four or five days on fresh fruit, such as grapefruit, with an enema each morning.

The finest herbal remedy to take during this four or five days on fruit is Bitter Root which grows among the mountains of Europe, 4-30 grains of the root can be taken morning and evening, or a tea can be made by boiling an ounce of the root in 1 pint of water for half an hour. After cooling and straining, take a wineglassful of the infusion on rising and retiring. After the four or five days on fruit, take up the light fish and salad diet as outlined.

While on this diet the following mixture made from dried herbs should be taken:

    2 oz. Poplar bark
    1 oz. Golden seal
    1 oz. Bitter root
    1 oz. Culvers root
    ½ oz. Capsicum

Simmer these in 3 pints of water until half is left. Cool, strain and store in a cool place. The dose is a wineglassful of the mixture three times daily after meals.

Jaundice

Catarrh or inflammation of the bile-ducts will prevent the flow of bile from the liver and gall-bladder into the intestine. When this happens the bile finds its way into the blood and causes the yellowish skin condition which is a symptom of jaundice. Usually the inflammation starts in the duodenum and then spreads to the bile-duct. This can happen as a result of a chill or in cases of vaccination fever.

If the cause is from vaccination then Thuja occidentalis should be taken. It is a really wonderful remedy for this condition especially if it is used homoeopathically. The 200 potency is best. Take one powder of this first thing on rising and do not repeat the dose until improvement in the condition has slowed down or stopped, when the dose may be repeated. The results of this in cases of vaccination fever which produce the symptoms of jaundice can be nothing short of miraculous. In other cases of jaundice adopt the four or five days on fresh fruit with the morning enema and then take to a light diet as outlined for cirrhosis of the liver.

While on this diet, which should be closely adhered to until all symptoms have vanished, the following mixture should be prepared from dried herbs:

2 oz. Dandelion root
1 oz. Circuma
1 oz. Barberry bark
1 oz. Agrimony
1 oz. Poplar bark

Boil these dried herbs in 5 pints of water for an hour. Cool and strain and add half a teaspoonful of cayenne pepper. The dose is a large wineglassful three or four times a day according to severity of symptoms. It is a good plan to begin each day with the juice of a fresh lemon in half a tumbler of warm water. Do not sweeten this juice.

Here is another good mixture for all liver disorders especially when there is any fever present. Take the following dried herbs:

1 oz. Wild Cherry bark
1 oz. Rhubarb root
1 oz. Prickly ash berries
1 oz. Pleurisy root
1 oz. Culvers root

Boil these in 4 pints of water for one hour. Cool and strain. Take a wineglassful of the mixture three times daily or four times if the symptoms are acute. The rhubarb will stimulate the gall ducts and help in the excretion of all bilious material. It has a soothing effect on the mucous membrane as well as being an astringent and will certainly help to eradicate catarrh which may be the cause of the inflammation.

In all cases of liver disorders make sure that dandelion leaves form a liberal part of the salad meals and other greens such as· endive. A dressing of lemon juice and olive oil will also be found of great help.

Gall-Bladder Disease

The gall-bladder is a pear-shaped vessel which

serves as a store for some of the bile from the liver. The bile, which is a most important digestive substance, is manufactured in the liver and leaves it by way of the hepatic duct to the common bile-duct and from there to the duodenum as explained earlier. Most of it, however, is collected in the gall-bladder where by loss of water it becomes concentrated.

It is when a meal has been taken that about 20 minutes afterwards the gall-bladder releases the bile into the duodenum where it meets and mixes with the food from the stomach. This mixture of food and digestive juices from the stomach is acid while the duodenum is normally alkaline.

The most common disorders of the gall-bladder are inflammation and gall stones. The catarrh which results from inflammation is known as cholecystitis and is most common in middle-aged persons who lead sedentary lives. It occurs more frequently in women than men and the fair, over-weight types are the most prone. Prolonged and chronic inflammation can lead to cholelithiasis (gall stones).

Causes: Lack of exercise and the eating of too much starchy and stodgy food are the prime causes. Various infections such as infected tonsils and bad teeth can, by way of the blood stream, also set up infection of the gall-bladder from these remote parts. The germs which often find their way into the gall-bladder are those which normally live in the healthy intestine, such as bacillus coli, where they are quite harmless.

The catarrh resulting from the inflammation which is caused by too much starch intake and little or no exercise is, as would be supposed, a very good breeding ground for all types of harmful bacteria and it is known that the germs of typhoid fever, for example, will continue to survive in the gall-bladder for many years after an attack. This chronic catarrh, if left untreated, will in time lead to gall stones.

Symptoms: The stomach always feels overloaded after eating, with discomfort and loss of appetite. There is pain at the right side of the abdomen below the ribs and often aching under the right shoulder blade. Constipation is another usual feature, with sickness and vomiting. General depression and a feeling of being chronically ill and always tired and listless will follow.

Treatment: The first essential is to remove the cause. The diet must be completely changed and before going on to a properly balanced diet which will prevent the recurrence of the disease, it is essential to first of all rid the body of the toxins which have caused the condition in the first place.

The very best way to do this is first to spend three days on a restrictive diet of fresh fruit and raw vegetables. The best fruit for this condition, as for liver disorders, is grapefruit, and two or three pounds of the fruit should be eaten daily split up into three meals. The first part of each meal should be raw salad of fresh lettuce, endive, celery, parsley, cress, dandelion leaves, etc., according to season, with grated carrot, turnip, swede, etc. On the first morning of this three day eliminative treatment a 1 pint enema should be taken using the gravity douche, the second morning a 2 pint enema and on the third morning a 3 pint enema. The water which should be at blood heat when taken into the colon shoud be held for at least half an hour.

On the fourth day the two food treatment should be undertaken. This consists of one bottle of pure lemon juice (about 26 fluid ounces) and the same amount of pure olive oil. At about 11 a.m. on the fourth day, after the enema has been taken first thing in the morning and nothing at all eaten, the two food treatment should be commenced. Every 15 minutes a tablespoonful each of the lemon juice and the olive oil shoud be taken. This is repeated every 15 minutes until the lemon juice and the olive oil are exhausted. *Do not stop the treatment if you feel sick. Persevere with this at all costs.*

Eat nothing else the whole day and on the fifth day commence another three days on the grapefruit and salad diet with the daily enemas. At the end of this time most conditions of catarrh will have cleared up and from then on a sensible balanced diet should be adopted. This ought to consist of a light breakfast of fresh fruit in season, always bearing in mind the great advantage of grapefruit in this particular condition. A slice of buttered wholemeal toast may also be had with this meal.

Lunch and the evening meal should form the main meals of the day and one of them should always be a good salad with fresh lean meat, grated cheese or fish. The other can be cooked, consisting of two green vegetables as in season and two root vegetables such as carrot and turnip with fresh lean meat or fish. Take eggs only in moderation and not more than two in any week. It is a good plan to have a first drink on rising in the morning of pure lemon juice in warm water. This should be made with the juice of one fresh lemon or a tablespoonful of pure lemon juice and it should be unsweetened.

Herbal Mixture

The following is the best mixture to take for these complaints. Take the following dried herbs:

> 2 oz. Dandelion root
> 2 oz. Stone root
> 2 oz. Eunoymin
> 2 oz. Leptandrin

Pour over these 2½ pints of boiling water and simmer until 1 pint is left. Allow to cool and strain. Take half a tumbler of the mixture three times daily after meals. Make this mixture fresh every two days or so and keep stored in a cool place.

One last important thing is this treatment of gall-bladder disease is to remember the need for regular exercise. Walking is extremely good but it must be regular. Walk five miles every day without fail. There are many other forms of exercise which can be undertaken according to age and, for younger people, these include running, swimming, horse riding (which will shake your liver up). The main thing is to make sure that whatever kind of exercise you undertake it is regular and not just something which happens once weekly on a Saturday afternoon in an energetic hour.

Diseases of the Urinary System

The urinary system comprises the kidneys, ureters, the bladder and the urethra.

The Kidneys
These are glands lying below the waist line at the back of the abdomen. They take care of waste material from the blood in the form of urine which, with excessive water, passes through the kidneys via the tubes called the ureters. In this way the urine reaches the bladder whence it is excreted by the urethra. Each kidney is enclosed in a fibrous capsule. The blood supply to the kidneys is by the renal artery and vein and at the top of each kidney is a small ductless gland called the adrenal.

Obviously if the kidneys are out of order this will affect the whole body either directly or indirectly since acid wastes which should have been excreted are perhaps re-absorbed into the body with quite harmful and far reaching results. For this, if for no other reason, it is a good thing even when well to refresh the kidneys from time to time with one or other of the marvellous herbal kidney tonics which can be so readily obtained and which can be so useful in prevention as well as in cure. Here is an

easy way to make tea which if taken for a day or
two, two or three times a year, will keep most
ordinary folk free from any chronic kidney
affections. Take the following dried herbs:

1 oz. Asparagus root
1 oz. Parsley root
1 oz. Celery root
1 oz. Fennel

Pour a pint of boiling water over these herbs in a
clean teapot. Allow to stand until cool and then
take a wineglassful of the mixture with a few
drops of lemon juice before each meal for two
or three days consecutively.

Do this every three months or so and you will
be very well insured against kidney disease later
in life. This tea, as will be seen, is made up of
herbs which are also culinary vegetables which
can be used whenever in season in salads or
properly cooked with any main meal. This will
afford added protection.

The strawberry root can also be added to this
tea, using 1 oz. of the root to the other four
herbs. It is not generally known, but the
strawberry, like the Willow Tree mentioned
earlier, is rich in natural salicin, and quite the
contrary to what is so often heard it is
extremely good in the treatment of rheumatism,
especially the inflammatory types.

When it is realized that uric acid and other
wastes of the urine such as sarcolactic acid are
often causes of rheumatism, and these wastes are
excreted by the kidneys, it can easily be seen
why the strawberry can not only be a good

kidney tonic but a very good way of avoiding the consequences of excessive uric acid, etc., in the system such as the various painful rheumatic complaints.

Kidney Disease

Stones or Calculi are quite a common disease of the kidneys and their presence may be undetected until such time as they begin to pass towards the bladder. The pain can be particularly violent during their passage through the ureter. In these cases the above tea should be made every two or three days and long drinks of it taken at frequent intervals until the stone has been naturally passed. Copious amounts of fluid must be taken throughout the treatment. One of the finest herbal mixtures for stones or calculi is the following made from dried herbs:

     1 oz. Dropwort
     1 oz. Poplar bark
     1 oz. Clivers
     1 oz. Buchu leaves
     1 oz. Tansy

Boil these for 20 minutes and then allow to cool before straining, after which, dissolve 2 oz. of gum arabic in the liquor. Take a wineglassful of this mixture three times daily between meals with 10 drops of oil of cubebs in each dose.

Bright's Disease

This is a chronic inflammation of the kidneys also known as Nephritis. Pain in this condition is usually felt at the back of the loins. One of the best herbal mixtures for this is to take the following dried herbs:

1 oz. Golden seal
1 oz. Buchu leaves
1 oz. Prickly ash
1 oz. Broom

Boil for 20 minutes in 4 pints of water. Allow to cool, and strain. Take a tumblerful of the mixture three or four times a day and make fresh supplies of this every two or three days.

Strangury

This complaint can have many causes such as inflammation in the kidneys, bladder or the urinary passages, or it may be caused by stones. There is a frequent urge to pass urine but this is always slow and painful and sometimes only a few drops can be passed at a time. Enlargement of the prostate gland in older men can also be a cause and this is dealt with later under the heading of 'prostate gland'.

When the cause is due to general inflammation, catarrh of the bladder, etc., use the following well tried and highly successful herbal mixture:

1 oz. Parsley piert
1 oz. Wild carrot
1 oz. Pelitory of the Wall
1 oz. Woodruff

Boil this for 20 minutes and allow to cool before straining, ready for use. Take half a tumbler of this mixture three times daily into which 10 drops of oil of juniper have been placed.

Suppression of Urine

This is a serious condition in which the kidneys fail to produce urine, usually as a result of acute inflammation sometimes due to fever, etc. Prompt treatment is essential if it is to be effective. Hot and cold compresses over the kidney region are very helpful.

To make a cold compress wring out a large handkerchief in cold water and place over the area. Place an old warm woollen garment over this and loosely hold in place. It should be kept on for up to two hours, when a sensation of warmth is experienced in the first 20 minutes. If this does not happen commence with a hot flannel compress for half an hour and then try the cold compress again.

Here is a well tried herbal mixture which should produce good results swiftly. Take the following dried herbs:

> 1 oz. Broom
> 1 oz. Dandelion root
> 1 oz. Tansy
> 1 oz. Pellitory
> ½ oz. Valerian

Simmer these in 4 pints of water until only half the quantity is left. A wineglassful of this mixture should be taken every two hours after it has been cooled and strained.

Retention of the Urine

This can be caused by a kind of paralysis following shock such as after an operation, etc., or by an obstruction such as stricture or stone or from an enlarged prostate gland. Vapour baths are very good for this condition, as are hot compresses of Camomile Flowers over the bladder region. To make such a compress, pour boiling water over a quantity of the flowers just enough to soak them well. Place these over the bladder area and cover with a piece of linen. Cover again with some old woollen garment and bind loosely. Leave on for one hour.

As an internal mixture make up the following dried herbs:

  2 oz. Slippery elm bark
  2 oz. Marshmallow root
  1 oz. Tansy
  1 oz. Juniper berries

Simmer these in 3 pints of water until only 2 pints are left. Strain and then add to the hot mixture 2 oz. of gum arabic, stirring until entirely dissolved. The dose is a wineglassful every three to four hours.

Enuresis

Enuresis, or involuntary flow of urine is often caused by chronic general debility, or paralysis. Sometimes there is no obvious cause. One of the most successful herbal mixtures for this embarrassing complaint is to take the following dried herbs:

  2 oz. Bistort root
  1 oz. White poplar
  1 oz. Valerian
  1 oz. Beth root

Simmer these in 4 pints of water until only 1 is

left. Cool and strain. The dose is a wineglassful of the mixture three times daily between meals. This will be found particularly useful for children who suffer from involuntary discharge of urine at night.

In all the above complaints when they are accompanied by burning sensations the famous Holborn Herbalist Gerard recommended an unguent made with the juice of cowslips and oil of linseed. This could be massaged into the bladder region and also across the small of the back.

It is interesting to know that Gerard, who is almost as famous as Culpeper in British Herbalism, was a neighbour of our famous Shakespeare and it is quite possible that these two were on visiting terms. How interesting it would be to know what conversation passed between these two — both great artists in their own particular field.

Women's Complaints

It is perhaps in the field of women's ailments that the surgeon during the last century has reaped his richest harvest. It would seem that the merest excuse has been needed in the past to operate and remove from countless thousands of women their organs of reproduction. Certainly surgery may be necessary in extreme cases and as a last resort but it is equally certain that a great deal of surgery could be obviated if the proper steps were taken at the right time and many so-called serious cases could be avoided by prompt and commonsense treatment along natural herbal lines.

On average, the allotted span of woman is some years longer than that of her male counterpart. She may not be so physically strong as man but she has much greater powers of endurance and suffering. The female of our species is designed to carry a greater burden and a greater physiological responsibility than the male. The supply of nutrition during the development of the embryo during pregnancy and the discomfort of carrying require a special temperament although this need not, as so many people imagine, involve greater suffering.

Indeed, childbirth and pregnancy can be free

from suffering, and if the childbirth is a natural one and the mother is fit and healthy then it will also be a painless one. Pregnancy is not a disease and does not, as so many people seem to think, require any special treatment. Our race has prospered and multiplied not because of but despite, the often barbarous regimens and treatments meted out to women during childbirth and labour.

The many species of life beside our own are able to multiply and thrive without any intellectual help and species only die out when interfered with and interrupted by influences outside them and beyond their control. They do not require the advice and attention of specialist gynaecologists. They can and do survive very well without them.

For a woman to have a comfortable and natural childbirth experience it is first essential to make sure that the ordinary everyday natural laws of living are observed. Diet is of primary importance with adequate exercises and plenty of fresh air.

A pregnant woman is not an invalid. In diet, account has to be taken of the growing foetus but this does not mean that the mother-to-be has to eat twice the amount of food in order to make sure that her baby is also receiving the right amount of nutrition for development. It does mean though, that the quality of the food is of the utmost importance if the child when it is born will commence life with the best possible chance of survival and of being able to grow and develop as a normal healthy individual in its own right.

As mentioned in the chapter on circulatory diseases, physiological iron is one of the great factors in a woman's health during pregnancy. This being so, make sure that each meal consists of fresh whole natural foods. If a mental resolution is made and carried out that no food, unless it conforms to the definition of being fresh and whole, will be eaten, then a great deal of needless suffering will be avoided and the mother-to-be can rest assured that her baby when it arrives will be sound and healthy with every possible chance of survival and of growing into a healthy balanced human being.

Suppressive drugs of any kind are not only unnecessary but are harmful and must be avoided at all costs. On the other hand the Herbalist can offer some plant extracts which will be of great help and which will promote a happy and painless childbirth. Among these are the raspberry leaf. A tea can be made from the dried leaves very easily and if this is taken regularly during pregnancy most women can look forward to a completely painless birth.

Take 2 oz. of the dried leaves obtained from any good Herbalist and simmer these in 1½ pints of boiling water for 20 minutes. Allow the whole to cool before straining ready for use. A wineglassful of the tea should be taken three or four times daily between meals during the whole period of pregnancy for the best results. Make a fresh supply of this tea every two days or so.

Never keep it too long.

Dropsy of the Womb

In the first stages this can often be confused with pregnancy. It can be caused by a blow or fall producing inflammation or may be the after effects of operative measures during delivery. The condition is accompanied by symptoms such as loss of appetite, some nausea, bearing down sensations and pain and swelling of the breasts as well as swelling and tenderness of the abdomen. The accumulated fluid can often be discharged from time to time, only to form again.

Treatment: For effective treatment it is essential to make sure that the skin is functioning properly and for this purpose hot and cold baths are desirable. Take a hot water bath of about five minutes duration followed by a tepid or cold shower every day on rising. Dry immediately with a good rough towel. The finest herbal treatments for this condition consist of tonics and bitters. One of the best mixtures can be made as follows from prepared dried herbs:

> 1 oz. Agrimony
> 1 oz. Clivers
> 1 oz. Burnett saxifrage
> 1½ oz. Dandelion roots

Place these in 4 pints of boiling water and gently simmer until 2 pints are left. Cool and then strain after which add a teaspoonful of cayenne. Take a wineglassful of the mixture every two hours until the symptoms subside after which reduce to four times daily until completely cured.

Another valuable mixture for this complaint is to take the following dried herbs:

1½ oz. Pellitory of the Wall
1½ oz. Broom
1 oz. Parsley piert
1 oz. Juniper berries
½ oz. Mountain flax

Add these to 5 pints of boiling water and gently simmer for an hour. When cold, strain and bottle for use. Take two tablespoonfuls of this mixture three times daily after meals.

Inflammation of the Womb

A chill during pregnancy or violent exercise, a sudden jolt such as during horse riding or dancing excessively, may produce inflammation of the womb. It may be the result of delivery and it can be acute or chronic. There may be some congestion present.

Treatment: Attention to hygiene is essential with plenty of fresh air and a psychologically cheerful approach to everyday affairs. The following should be prepared and the mixture taken until the symptoms have cleared up:

1 oz. Marshmallow root
1 oz. Chamomile flowers
1 oz. Lady's slipper

Place these prepared herbs in 2 pints of boiling water and simmer gently for half an hour. Allow to cool and then strain. Take half a tumblerful of the mixture three times daily between meals.

Prolapsus (Dropped Womb)

This often happens after childbirth especially if the diet has not been sound and there is loss of elasticity in the tissues. Another symptom of this loss of elasticity is varicose veins when they appear after childbirth and which are dealt with in the chapter on circulation. If the ligaments which hold the womb in place lose their elasticity the womb will drop. Another cause can be undue strain which causes the ligaments to become relaxed.

Symptoms: Pain will be experienced in the small of the back and in the groins. This pain will be aggravated by standing or walking for any length of time. There is a sensation of bearing down — a dull, heavy, wearing pain. There will be pressure on the bladder and the rectum which may cause symptoms of difficulty in urination and constipation. The severity of these symptoms will naturally vary with the degree and extent of the prolapse.

Treatment: In order to alleviate the symptoms as early as possible, hip baths should be introduced at once. The patient should sit in about five inches of cold water for two minutes first thing on rising and again on retiring every day for two or three weeks. After the immersion, dry thoroughly with a warm towel. This will stimulate and strengthen the tissue, helping to tone up the relaxed ligaments.

A cold compress round the waist at night is a good alternative to the hip baths. For this a band of linen about six inches wide and long enough to go round the body should be wrung out in cold water and placed round the hips. This should then be wrapped round with an old woollen garment large enough to completely encircle the waist. This should be pinned and left in position all night, if warmth is felt after five minutes or so. If warmth is not generated it should be removed and tried again on a subsequent night and if not successful, adopt the hip bath treatment.

When loss of elasticity is due to inadequate nutrition during pregnancy and there are also symptoms of varicose veins the wonderful comfrey root should be taken over a long period. For this it is advisable to obtain a supply of the manufactured liquid extract from a qualified Registered Medical Herbalist. A drachm of this extract should be taken three times daily after meals for several months.

A very good and reliable herbal mixture which can be prepared at home and which can have wonderful results in this condition is to take the following dried herbs:

    1½ oz. Collinsonin (stone root)
    1 oz. Comfrey root
    1 oz. White poplar
    1 oz. Oak bark

Place these in 4 pints of boiling water and simmer until about half is left. Cool and strain and take half a tumblerful of the mixture three times daily after meals.

Dysmenorrhoea (Painful Menstruation)

This is one of the most common complaints with which women have to live. It can occur at any time from puberty to the 'change of life'. It can be the result of many causes such as inflammation of the womb, rheumatism, chills, strain, or it can be the result of psychological disturbances brought about by grief, worry or over-excitement.

Symptoms: These are pain, usually two or three days before discharge, in the loins, in the small of the back as well as the abdomen. Sometimes pain is experienced in the thighs. There is a feeling of faintness, sometimes nausea, with headaches and neuralgia and the patient becomes very irritable. Sometimes during the menstrual period the blood will discharge in clots and if left untreated these symptoms will become of longer duration with each succeeding period.

Treatment: The hot and cold water treatments are very effective in this condition and the same procedure should be followed as outlined for prolapsus. Steam or turkish baths will also be found most useful in alleviating the painful symptoms, while the most useful herbal mixture can be prepared from the following dried herbs:

    1 oz. Ground pine
    1 oz. Southernwood
    1 oz. Tansy
    1 oz. Catmint

Place these in 4 pints of boiling water and

simmer until about 2 pints are left and pour the boiling liquor from the residue of herbs on to one ounce of black cohosh. Allow this to cool and then strain. Take a wineglassful of the mixture four times daily between meals.

Menorrhagia (Flooding or profuse menstruation)
This is an excessive bleeding from the womb and can happen at any time and at any age. It can have a variety of causes. If flooding happens during pregnancy it is usually a sign of a threatened miscarriage. It can be the result of a congenital abnormality of the womb or it can happen immediately or a few days after childbirth when it is often due to part of the afterbirth remaining in the womb with a consequent prevention of the normal process of the sealing up of the blood vessels. Again it can occur at the 'change of life' and in fact it is a quite common phenomenon at this time. At the other end of the scale it can happen at puberty when menstruation is just commencing.

Treatment: In the case of flooding after childbirth it is essential first to empty the womb as soon as possible of anything that may have been left so that there shall be no chance of blood poisoning. Massage of the abdomen to affect the womb with infusion of oak bark can be very beneficial. Here are two wonderful herbal mixtures for this complaint which are always helpful. Take the following prepared dried herbs:

1 oz. Cudweed
1 oz. Cranesbill
1 oz. Beth root
1 oz. Unicorn root

Place these in 4 pints of boiling water and simmer until 3 pints are left when the mixture should be allowed to stand and cool before straining ready for use. The dose is half a tumblerful of the mixture three times daily after meals. The alternative mixture can be made as follows with dried herbs:

1 oz. Bistort root
1 oz. Tortmentil root
1½ oz. Beth root

Place these in 3 pints of boiling water and simmer gently until 2 pints are remaining. After allowing to cool, strain and the mixture is ready for use. The dose is the same as for the first mixture, half a tumblerful three times daily after meals.

Amenorrhoea (Suppressed Menstruation)

The causes of suppressed menstruation can be many and various. Chills, colds, fevers, anaemia, general debility as well as mental strains and stresses can be predisposing factors. Worry, shock, psychological disturbances and in fact a host of general factors can cause or contribute to the cause of this condition.

Symptoms: Menstruation always ceases in a natural way during pregnancy and during lactation. It ceases again in a natural way at the commencement of the menopause (change of life). When not due to natural causes, the main symptoms are often anaemia, loss of weight, headaches, rheumatic pains in the back and down the limbs, loss of appetite, inflammation of the womb and a general listlessness.

Treatment: Massage to the lumbar region has been found very beneficial, and sitz baths or the abdominal cold compress treatment as outlined earlier are also helpful. The finest herbal treatment which often produces wonderful results quite quickly is to take the following dried herbs:

> 2 oz. Motherwort
> 1 oz. Golden seal
> 1 oz. Chamomile
> 1 oz. Blue cohosh
> ½ oz. Ginger

Place these herbs in 4 pints of boiling water and gently simmer until 2 pints remain. Allow to cool and then strain prior to use. The dose is half a tumblerful of the mixture three times daily after meals. At the same time it is essential to see that the diet is adequate in such foods as eggs, lean meat and fish.

Leucorrhoea (The Whites)

This is a very common and distressing condition and can occur at almost any age and at any time. It consists of a discharge usually from the vagina although it can come from the womb and is of a whitish colour. It can be a symptom of more serious disease or can result from lack of cleanliness. In children it can be a symptom of threadworms or some other irritation. It can be due to weakness and debility.

Treatment: Cleanliness is essential and the vagina should be washed out daily with soothing and cleansing antiseptics. A good douche can be made by taking the following extracts obtained from a good Herbalist:

2 oz. Fluid extract of Hydrastis
8 oz. Distilled extract of Witch Hazel

Mix these together and use an ounce of the mixture to a pint of water at blood heat for the douche, and wash the parts thoroughly twice daily. A very reliable herbal treatment which should soon clear the condition is to take the following dried herbs:

1 oz. Golden seal
1 oz. Prickly ash
1 oz. Solomon's seal
½ oz. Unicorn root

Place these in 3 pints of boiling water and simmer gently until about 1 pint is left. Cool and strain ready for use. The mixture should be taken in doses of a wineglassful three times daily after meals.

Menopause (Change of Life)

This usually occurs in women between the ages of 40 and 50 and should be quite natural in character and without any untoward symptoms. However, due to the stresses and strains of modern living, with poor diet and other causes, it can sometimes be accompanied by symptoms which become distressing. The periods become scantier and often miss some months when they are due, before ceasing altogether.

This is usually quite normal and can continue for about two years. Sometimes there are symptoms of flushing (a rush of blood to some part of the body) with palpitations and hot sweats followed by feelings of chill and cold. These frequently happen at night, and can be quite unpleasant experiences. All kinds of nervous symptoms can also make their appearance. Neuralgic pains often appear and disappear without warning and there is also a tendency to put on weight. For this the diet must be watched carefully. Most women pass through this period without harm. Others suffer very much and for these the finest herbal treatment is as follows:

     1 oz. Golden seal
     1 oz. Pulsatilla
     1 oz. Motherwort
     1 oz. Tansy
     1 oz. Black haw
     ½ pz. Arrach

Simmer these in 3 pints of boiling water until about 2 pints are left. Cool and strain. Take half a tumblerful of the mixture in as much water three times daily between meals. This mixture should be taken over a period of several months or even a year.

Conclusion

Naturally in a small book of this limited scope it is only possible to deal with the more common ailments to which women are prone and in all cases of serious symptoms it cannot be too strongly stressed that the sufferer should seek and follow the advice of a Registered Medical Herbalist where more specialized and individual treatment can be obtained.

Some Useful Information

In the preceding chapters of this handbook the body has been split into its main systems and really sound constructive treatments of a purely natural character have been presented which, if used properly and according to the instructions, will bring about remarkable results. In addition, some of the principal organs have been dealt with and the afflictions to which they are most prone.

The treatments have all been devised in such a way that they can be carried out in the home and all the mixtures recommended can be prepared by anyone. Every herb mentioned can be obtained quite easily from any good retail Herbalist. The more rare and costly herbs have been purposely left out and all the mixtures used are in the form of easily made decoctions. No specialist knowledge is therefore necessary either in the reading of this book or in the preparation of any of the recommended prescriptions.

Herbal medicine has a secure place in the treatment of disease and because new and quick acting drugs are always being discovered is no reason to discard and ignore what has been proved and found effective over countless hundreds of years. These remedies are just as effective today in the alleviation of cure of disease as ever they were and readers of this book who really follow the advice and instruction herein will be fully rewarded in renewed health and vigour and what is equally important, the fear of chronic and incurable disease will disappear.

This section deals with one or two conditions which are not covered in the previous sections and which are quite common in occurrence. They cannot be properly included in the various divisions of the systems of the body which are dealt with nor do they come ordinarily under the disease conditions of the organs mentioned. They are nonetheless important, especially to those who may be sufferers. Conditions of the thyroid gland and the prostate are sufficiently common to warrant attention and treatments are given in the following pages for conditions of these glands as well as for other fairly common complaints which can be treated privately in the home.

Thyroid Conditions

An upset of this gland can have far reaching effects on the whole system. Its hormone secretion is vital to the health of the whole body and it is intimately concerned with individual vitality. It can be responsible for such seemingly remote ailments as stomach upsets and intestinal complaints. It can effect the eyes. Again the Herbalist relies on that wonderful remedy previously mentioned — the Primrose — for all conditions caused by disorders of the thyroid gland. The instructions for using this as an infusion or decoction should be followed in all cases where the thyroid may be responsible. It can have nothing short of miraculous results.

The Prostate Gland

Many men find their lives made a misery in middle and later life by inflammation of this gland. It can enlarge and cause the retention of urine or so impede its excretion as to cause many complications from the presence of this toxic waste for too long in the bladder.

If only the virtues of Saw Palmetto were better known in this respect it is certain there would be a lot fewer prostate sufferers. Most Herbalists know of its wonderful effect on all glandular tissues but it has a special affinity for the prostate. It is best obtained from your Herbalist as a liquid extract and a dose of 10-25 minims taken three or four times daily between meals.

It is not generally known, but this herb will also help to build up fresh young healthy tissue in underweight individuals. It is, in fact, a wonderful nutrient of the body. Certainly anyone suffering from disorders of the prostate can expect to obtain really remarkable results by taking this herb; 15 grains of the powdered berries may be taken as an alternative to the liquid extract.

In cases where this trouble is accompanied by

sexual impotency it can be combined with Damiana and Kola nut; 1 oz. of each of the dried herbs simmered in two pints of water until one pint is left. Cool, strain and take a wineglassful of the mixture after meals.

Another herb which can be used in this respect is Sarsaparilla. It is not generally known but this herb contains the equivalent of the male hormone testosterone. Together with Sassafras it can be made into a pleasant tea and will maintain vitality and prevent all kinds of middle-age complaints such as rheumatism.

Rheumatic Complaints

We all know that the orthodox profession use the drug cortisone for the treatment of arthritis and this is made from the testes of the bull containing the hormone. How much better and safer to use a plant remedy which contains the male hormone testosterone in these ailments where the vital ingredients are maintained by nature in correct proportion to one another. Certainly no shocking side effects will ever be experienced by taking Sarsaparilla Root.

A word about Sarsaparilla. This grows mainly in America, India and Jamaica. Although from whatever origin they all have similar properties, by far the best variety is that grown in Jamaica. Herbalists use this root with Sassafras and other famous herbs such as Blue flag, Burdock and Queen's delight with immense success in all types of rheumatic disease. Here is one of the best combinations of these herbs to make up for yourself:

Take of the following dried herbs 1 oz. of each Jamaican Sarsaparilla, Queen's delight, Burdock, Poke root and Blue flag and simmer them in 3 pints of water until 2 pints are left. Cool and strain for use. Take a wineglassful after every meal and enjoy a good anti-rheumatic tonic. Far better than the artificial stimulants so readily taken in huge quantities these days.

The Hair

Many people suffer with disorders of the hair; falling hair, premature greyness, etc. This is often an indication that the general health is at fault. Hair is an excretion of the body and consists of almost pure protein. First look to the diet in all these conditions and make sure than an adequate amount of good protein food is included. Make sure this reaches the scalp by regular daily moving of the scalp on the skull. NOT just rubbing the hair; this is useless.

A wonderful herbal help to the health of the hair is to mix an ounce of oil of rosemary with an ounce of oil of sage and gently massage this into the roots of the hair about an hour before washing the hair. It should then be washed with a rosemary shampoo which can be obtained from any Health Food Store. When thoroughly dry use a lotion of Rosemary Hair Tonic, (also obtainable from any Health Food Store) every day to encourage growth and health.

A Healthy Skin

There are so many skin foods and other preparations on the market that it may seem superfluous to mention any more but among the wonderful herbals we have is one which can be relied on to keep the skin in good condition and to preserve its youthfulness and stave off that time when wrinkles arrive round the eyes, etc.

A cream made from Calendula is the ideal. It can be used also as a lotion and this can be made at home by boiling 2 oz. of dried cut Calendula in 1 pint of water for 20 minutes. Cool and strain and keep in a cool place for nightly application as a lotion for the face. Allow to dry on the skin. Calendula skin cream is obtainable from all the well known Herbalists.

Care of the Eyes

This is something which is often ignored until sight is impaired or the eye muscles become weak and glasses have to be resorted to. Daily use of the well known herbal Eyebright as an eye bath will often avoid this and assist in the maintenance of good sight throughout life. Eyebright or Euphrasia as it is known by its Latin name can be prepared at home. It is useful as an internal medicine as well as an eye lotion.

The juice of the Eyebright can be used as eye drops. It can be combined with that wonderful remedy of which we spoke earlier in this book to make a really excellent lotion for strengthening the eyesight. It can be obtained ready made for use with an eye bath from most Health Food

Stores and Herbalists.

Spongy or Bleeding Gums, Pyorrhoea

This seems to be a very common ailment in these days. Before any lasting cure can be obtained the diet must be modified to include adequate amounts of Vitamin C and this means plenty of fresh fruit.

Eating apples is one of the finest helps to healthy teeth and gums. The finest way to clean the teeth and stimulate the gums is to eat at least one apple after every meal. For a good herbal treatment we turn again to Calendula which can have a wonderful effect on the most chronic cases of bleeding gums. For this the tincture is required and this should be held in the mouth for two or three minutes every morning on rising and again on retiring. Just a teaspoonful is enough and it can be put into a small quantity of water for this purpose.

Conclusion

Although in recent years many new, so-called wonder drugs, have been foisted on to the public as great advances in the treatment and cure of many classes of disease there is no doubt at all that the old herbal remedies are still the most useful and efficacious. When used with proper knowledge and if persevered with they can do nothing but good and the range of application and action of these plants ensures that all chronic sufferers can turn to nature's dispensary with renewed hope.

Many a chronic sufferer near to despair has found relief and cure among this wide range of nature's products which are there for the collecting. It must be remembered that man in his original state was completely herbivorous, and it logically follows that even now after so many hundreds of years drifting away from this once ideal diet he could do worse than seek among these wonderful weeds the things that will help in times of illness and distress.

Other books for better health the natural way.

LIVING WITH ANGINA
R. William Thompson

Written by an angina sufferer, this book explains how to cope with the illness and live as full a life as possible. It describes the workings of the heart and how angina is caused, and the method of treatment by diet and relaxation which has helped the author. It also shows how the angina patient can adapt his working and home conditions for maximum activity and independence, and how his family can best deal with the situation.

ARTHRITIS
Help In Your Own Hands
Helen B. MacFarlane

The story of one woman's successful fight against crippling arthritis, and how she regained full use of her limbs by a combination of diet, special exercises and massage. With notes on aids and appliances available for all arthritis sufferers.

MOLASSES AND NUTRITION
Alan Moyle, N.D., M.B.N.O.A.

Explains the nutritional significance of molasses and its value in treating many disorders, including constipation, intestinal troubles and rheumatism; with an account of sugar cane harvesting and a varied selection of molasses recipes for laxative mixtures, muesli, puddings, cakes, jellies and scones.

HERBAL TEAS
For Health and Healing
Ceres

Herbal teas, apart from being much better for you than the Indian or China teas which are so popular, make delicious drinks and can 'dispel all manner of discomforts'. The author — lifelong naturalist, broadcaster and contributor to *The Times* — describes over a hundred herbs and gives instructions for making and using the teas.

PROVEN REMEDIES
J.H. Oliver N.A.M.H.

Herbs and plants contain healing properties which can benefit the ailing without the injurious side effects associated with drugs. Such 'proven remedies' consist of biochemic, botanic, herbal and homoeopathic preparations which the author prescribes for a large number of alphabetically listed ailments.

HERBS FOR COLDS AND 'FLU
Nalda Gosling F.N.I.M.H.

Describes twenty-one herbs most helpful in treating colds and 'flu, and for minimizing or eliminating subsequent catarrh, cough or bronchial conditions. Includes herbs for restoring normal appetite and banishing the lethargy and depression associated with 'flu.

HERBS AND FRUIT FOR VITAMINS
Ceres

Explains the vitamin content of alfalfa, apricot, bistort, buckwheat, couch grass, cowslip, dandelion, lungwort, sunflower, tomato, and other herbs and fruit, with suggestions for their use as interesting and healthful dietary additions.

THE SLIMMER'S GUIDE TO CALORIES
R. Newman Turner N.D., D.O.

An explanation in human terms of what calories are, their function, and how to control them for the purpose of losing weight. Provides tables which enable the reader to select lower calorie foods without sacrificing an element of choice.

YOUR DIET IN HEALTH AND DISEASE
Harry Benjamin N.D.

A complete explanation of the food we eat, its relationship to the health or disease of our bodies, and how to digest, absorb and assimilate it. Includes a self-treatment chart for common ailments.